26 SIMPLE AND EFFECTIVE ABDOMINAL CORE EXERCISES

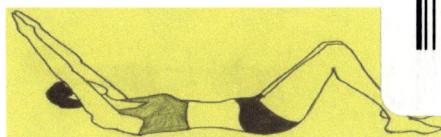

With Personalized sample workout.
Perform in your own home, at your convenience.

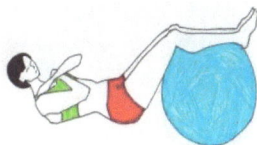

Illustrations by Gillian Marcus.

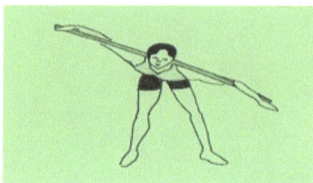

Work at your own pace.

A small investment of 10-20 minutes a day will change your life.

A Note to the Reader:

The exercises in this book are based on the author's personal research and practical application as a certified personal trainer. It is meant as a guide to provide instructions to the reader for safe and effective abdominal training workouts. The author disclaims all liability in connection with the use of the information in individual cases. Please consult your doctor about the suitability of exercises.

GET YOUR ABS ON

Simple and effective abdominal exercises designed to improve definition strengthen the core muscles and improve posture.

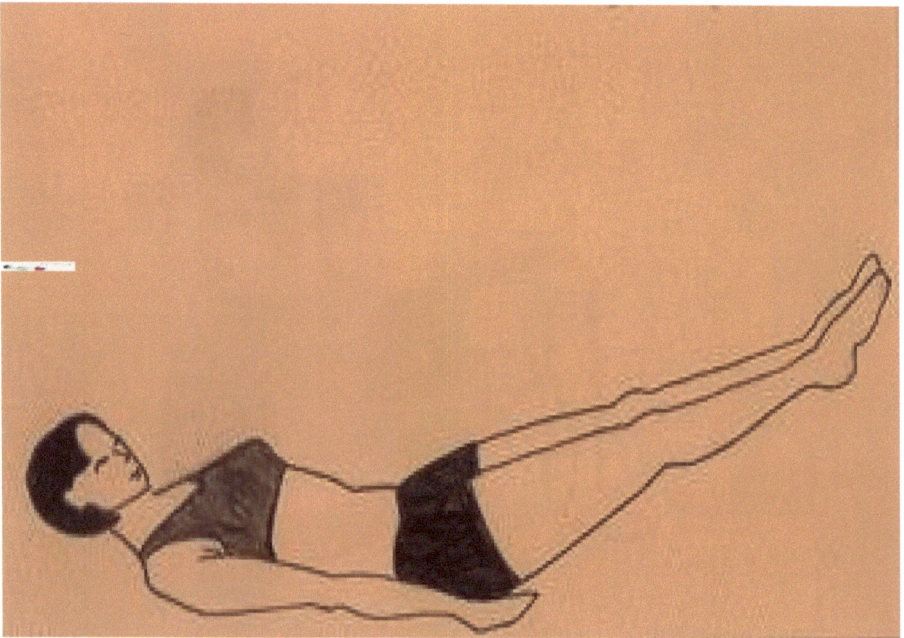

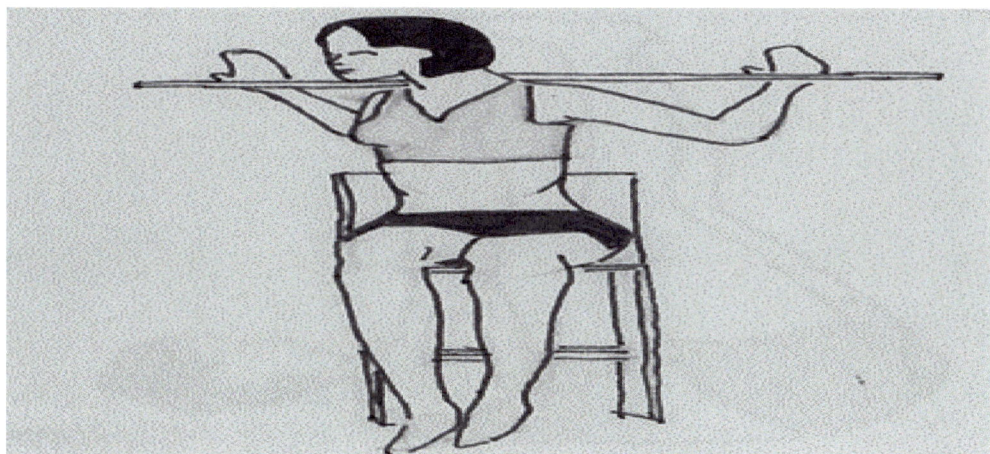

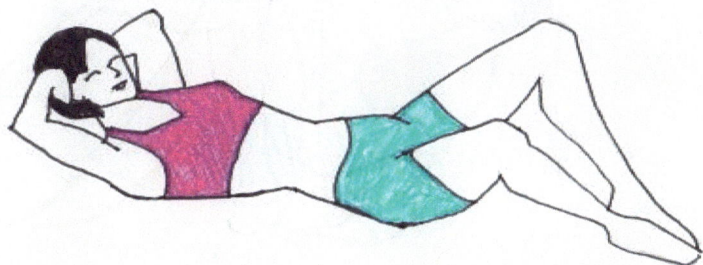

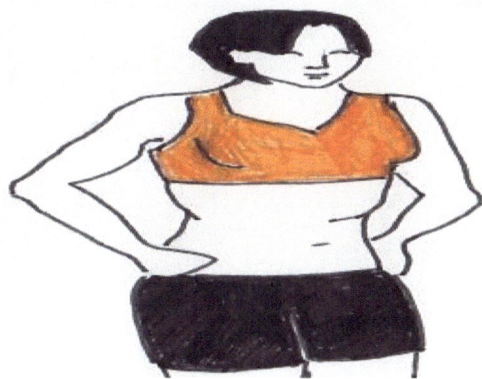

CONTENTS

Introduction

If you are anything, anything at all like me, you've been wondering for some time, "where did my abs go?" All is not lost! There is no time like the present to get started and GET YOUR ABS ON.

Abs are tricky little things – they tend to go in one direction or another, can expand or contract, AND, to put it very bluntly, the expansion part is quick and decisive, that is, it doesn't take very long to develop a beer belly.

So, it begs the question, why are abdominals so hard to define? What's the secret to well-defined abdominals? **Training and Nutrition! Train Abs Smart!** The worst thing you can do when training the abs is to do it mindlessly. Smart exercise
selection is crucial for getting the best results.

The benefits of having a set of highly developed abdominals are improved definition and better posture because the abdominals help keep the back straight. Overall health will also improve as training helps keep the internal organs in great functioning condition with all the blood being pumped into the training region.

The superficial muscle group of the midsection is the rectus abdominis which originates at the pubic crest at the front of the hips. It extends upward to insert on the ribcage and the lower part of the sternum (this is the muscle that makes up the entire waist) and covers the anterior part of the waist. The major muscles at the sides of the waist are the external obliques, serratus and intercoastals. Each of these muscles must be exercised separately to develop them equally.

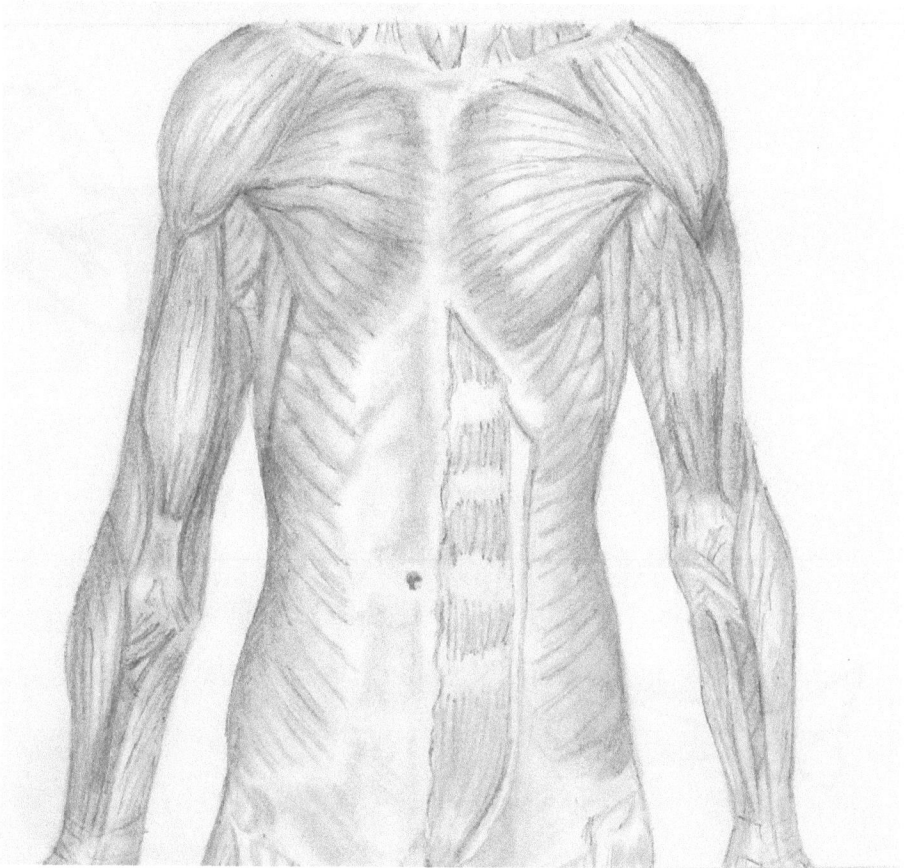

The lower abdominals are the most stubborn and exercise-resistant area, and many people consider this area the most difficult to define.

Just like all the other muscles of the body, the rectus abdominis (muscle responsible for abdominal rows) is developed when we challenge it to move against opposition greater than that to which it is accustomed.

Abs Exercise Tips and Myths

First of all, there is no such thing as "spot reduction." Doing thousands of abdominal crunches will tone the stomach muscles but won't eliminate the body fat that covers them. Abs training combined with twenty minutes of cardio training in your target heart range three times a week will go a long way towards reducing the adipose fat covering the belly.

Keep your lower back pushed into the floor, mat or bench. Try to imagine your shoulders pinned down to the mat. The act of pulling the wings of the shoulder blades down involves pressing the shoulder blades further down than their normal resting position in your upper back. This motion of depressing the shoulders or sliding them down and back will simultaneously lengthen the neck, strengthen the back and help alleviate neck and shoulder tension.

The proper position for abdominal exercises is to lengthen your spine along the mat and concentrate on pulling the navel in as you contract the abdominal muscles. As you keep the neck long and shoulders pinned down, try not to arch your back up. If you find in general that your back arches up, keep your knees bent and closer to your body so your lower back is pushing into the floor.

As you crunch up and forward, be sure that your head, neck and shoulder blades lift off the mat. Make sure you are not pulling your head forward with your hands. Keep your chin tucked in though it should not be making contact with your chest.

Train your lower abdominals first as they usually are the most difficult and will tire you faster. Breathe out as you crunch up. Remember, crunches isolate and train the abdominal muscles in a way no exercise equipment ever could.

So, *HAPPY CRUNCHING*!

UPPER ABS

1. Basic Abdominal Crunch

2. Crunch Hands Overhead

3. Crunch Legs on the Exercise Ball

4. Weighted Ball Crunches

5. Twisting Ball Crunches

6. Crossover Crunches

7. Frog Leg Crunches

8. Straight Leg Crunches

Basic Abdominal Crunch

Place your feet on the floor or mat with your heels comfortably away from your buttocks. Knees and hips should be bent at right angles.

Gently place your hands at your sides or behind your head.

Keep your elbows slightly out to the sides.

Lift your upper body slowly elevating your shoulder blades off the floor and crunching your rib cage towards your knees similar to a U-shaped position.

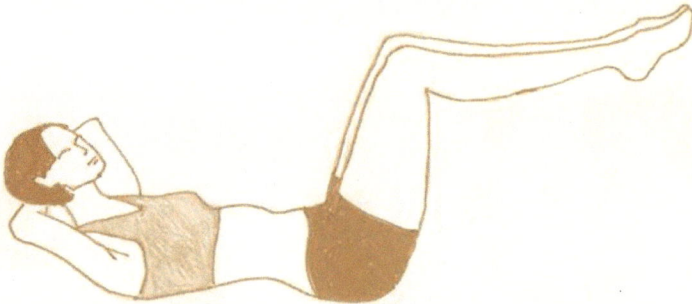

Your shoulders and mid-back should be off the floor.

Hold for a slow count of one to three at the top position then lower slowly to the starting position.

Begin the next rep immediately.

Don't rest between reps.

Perform 10-20 repetitions.

Crunch Hands Overhead

To increase the level of difficulty from the regular crunch, lie on the floor with your knees bent and feet flat on the floor.

Extend your arms overhead. Upper arms should be close to the ears then cross your palms.

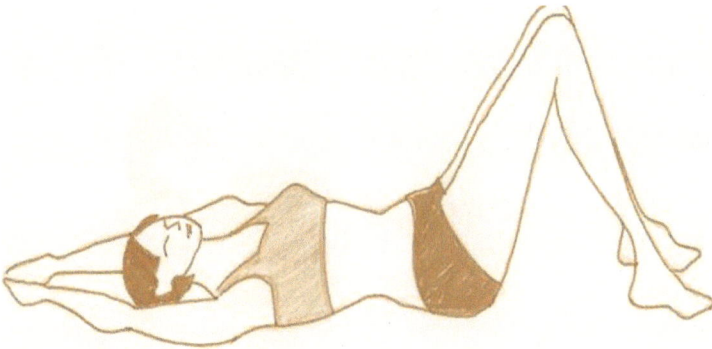

Curl your body forward lifting your shoulder blades first off the floor and deeply contracting the abs.

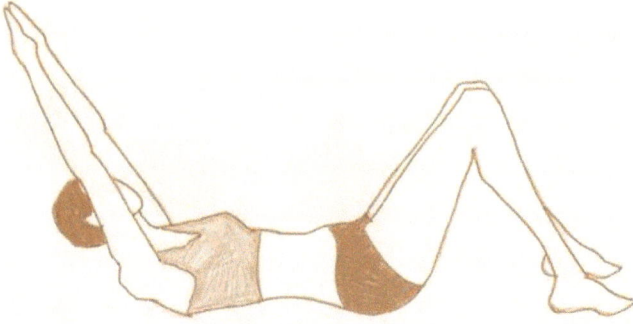

Keep your head level throughout.

Hold the top position for a slow count of one to three before lowering slowly down.

Perform 10-20 repetitions.

Crunch Legs on the Exercise Ball

Lie on the floor with your feet on a Swiss exercise ball about three inches apart.

Toes are turned inward.

Knees and hips are bent at right angles.

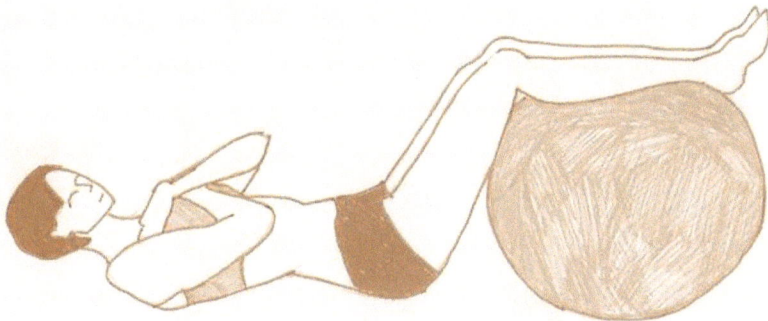

With arms crossed or hands on either side of the head crunch up.

Bring your shoulders up while lower back remains rooted to the floor.

Head remains level. Stabilize the ball.

Hold the top position for a slow count of one to three before lowering slowly down.

Perform 10-20 repetitions.

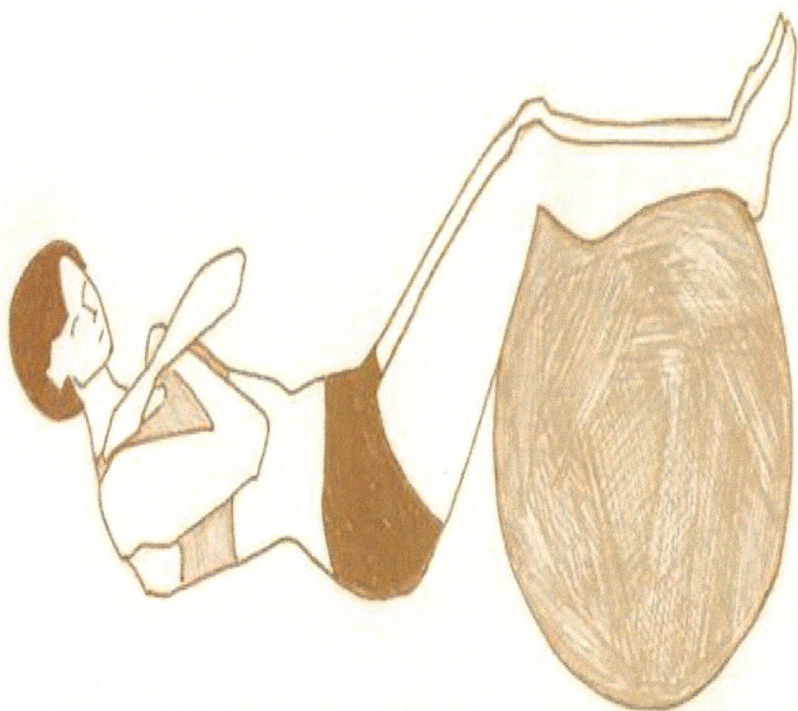

Weighted Ball Crunches

Lie back on the Swiss ball so the lower back is curled in and slightly elevated over the top of the ball.

Place your feet flat on the floor. Stabilize the ball.

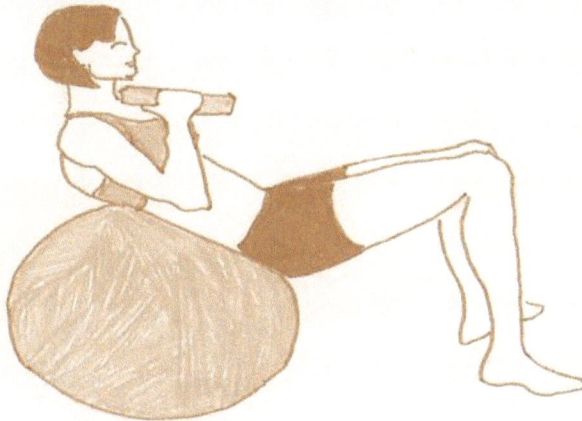

Using both hands, hold a 5lb dumbbell on the chest to begin.

Crunch up slowly using the shoulders while your lower back remains pressed into the ball.

Hold the top position for a slow count of one to three before lowering slowly down.

Perform 10-20 repetitions.

Twisting Ball Crunches

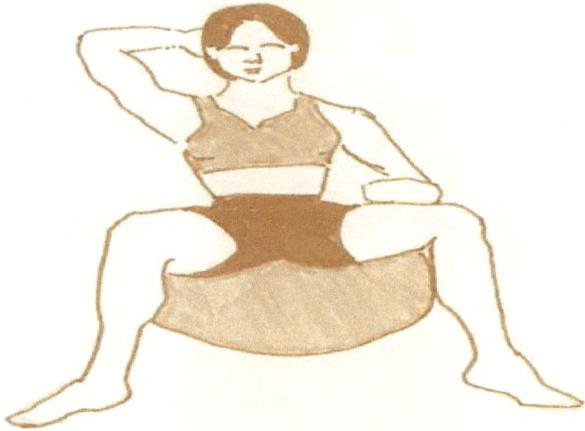

As in the previous exercise, lie back on the Swiss ball so the lower back is curled and slightly elevated over the top of the ball.

Place your feet flat on the floor. Stabilize the ball.

With your right hand at the back of the head and left hand at the waist, curl the shoulders up slowly.

Contract the abdominals and twist your upper body moving the right arm up and across the midline of the body.

Hold the top position for a slow count of one to three before lowering slowly down.

Perform 10-20 repetitions, and then switch sides. Complete two sets per side.

Crossover Crunches

Place your hand behind your head and position your right leg across your left knee.

Flex your abs before beginning the exercise and push your lower back into the floor.

Aim your right elbow towards your left knee, twist your entire torso and slowly breathe out.

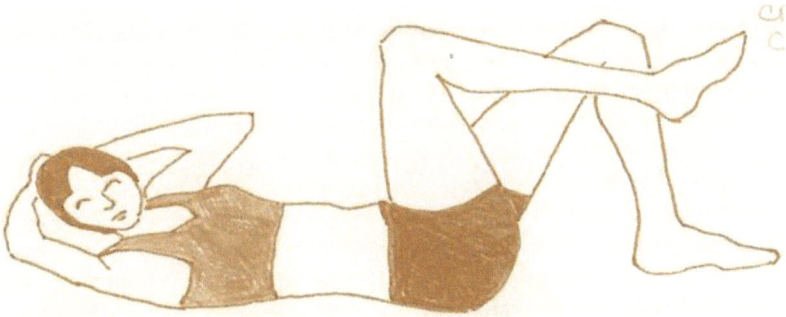

Contract your abs for two to three counts at the top of the movement. Slowly lower to starting position.

Perform 10-15 repetitions then switch sides.

Frog Leg Crunches

Lie on your back and bring the soles of your feet together.

Keeping the feet on the floor and knees to the sides, clasp your hands behind your head or cross the arms over the chest.

Using your upper abs, raise your shoulders and upper back off the floor, rolling the upper torso forward while keeping your lower back pressed against the floor.

Pause briefly at the top and lower the shoulders back slowly to the starting position.

Repeat when the shoulders touch the floor lightly.

Stay at a controlled speed.

Perform 10-20 repetitions.

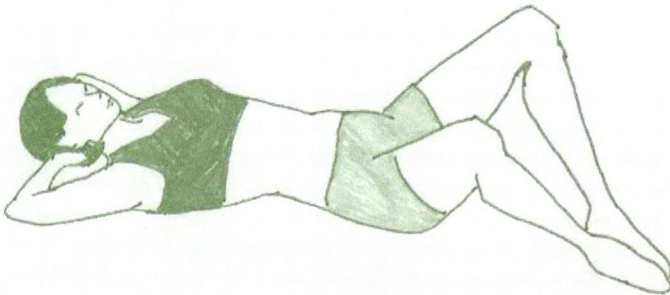

Straight Leg Crunches

Lie on your back with straight legs lifted perpendicular to the floor.

Clasp your hands behind your head.

With legs remaining stationary, use the upper abs to lift the shoulders off the floor.

Hold the top of the movement for two-counts and lower yourself back down.

Repeat once the shoulder blades touch the floor lightly.

Keep the small of the back pressed against the floor.

Don't raise the hips.

Use a controlled movement.

Perform 10-20 repetitions.

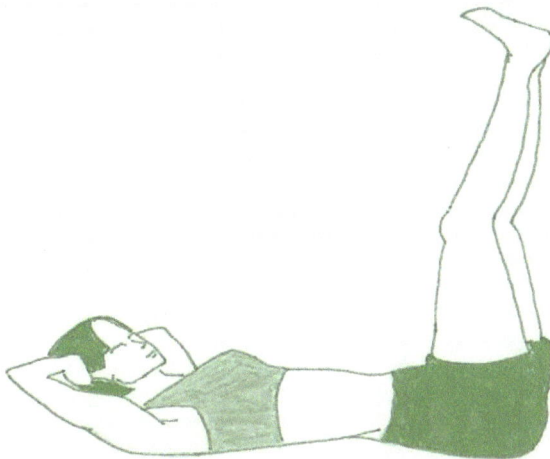

LOWER ABS

1. Knee-Ups

2. Scissor Kick

3. Leg Pull-In

4. Reverse Crunches

5. Lying Leg lifts

6. Jackknife Crunches

7. Hanging Leg Raises

Knee-Ups

Sit on the end of a bench or on the floor and lean back at about 45 degrees. Arms are extended along the sides.

Use your arms to stabilize your body.

Keep a slight bend in the knees and hold the feet just off the surface.

Contract the abs to pull your knees up towards your chest bending the legs as you do so while simultaneously curling your torso forward and contracting your abdominals.

Hold for a two-three second count at the top of the movement and return the legs slowly to a straightened position.

Perform 10-20 repetitions.

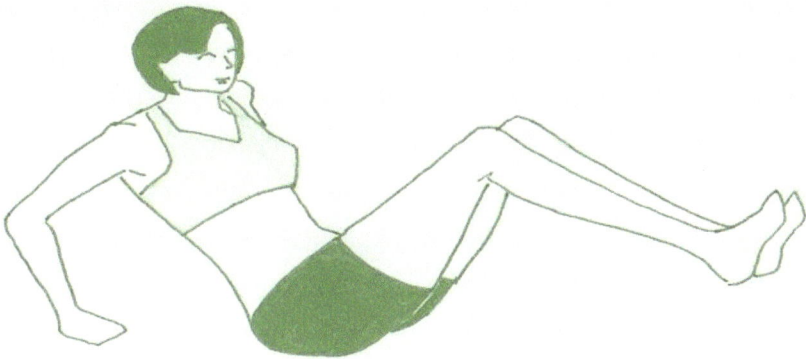

Scissor Kick

Lie on your back with your arms by your sides and your palms facing down.

Extend your legs fully with a slight bend in the knees and hold the feet about 6 inches off the floor.

Lift the right leg up while the left leg is lowered until the heel is about 3 inches from the floor.

Make rapid up and down scissor-like movements as you contract the abdominals with the lower back pressed into the mat.

Switch movements as your raise your left leg and lowering your right, lifting each leg to about 45 degrees into the air and lowering your heel to about 3 inches off the floor.

Perform 10-20 repetitions.

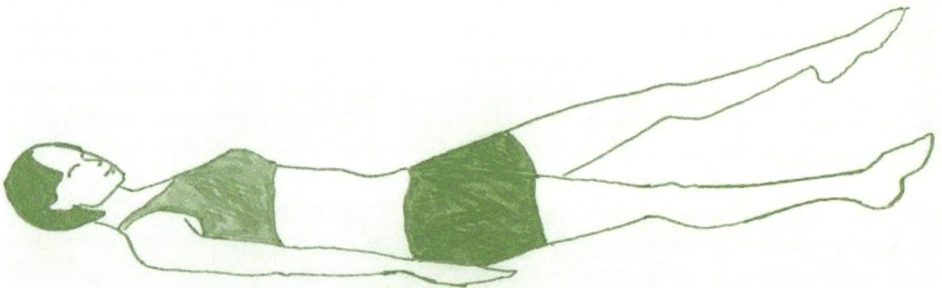

Leg Pull-In

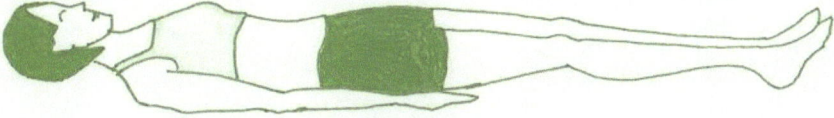

Lie on the floor, arms by your sides, your palms down legs extended straight along the floor.

As you inhale, lift your back off the floor, contract the abs bending your knees and bringing the legs close to the body pulling your thighs into your mid-section.

Rotate your pelvis forward to really crunch your abs.

Squeeze your abs at the top concentrating on your lower abdominals while keeping your legs together.

Remember slow and controlled! Try not to swing!

Perform 10-20 repetitions.

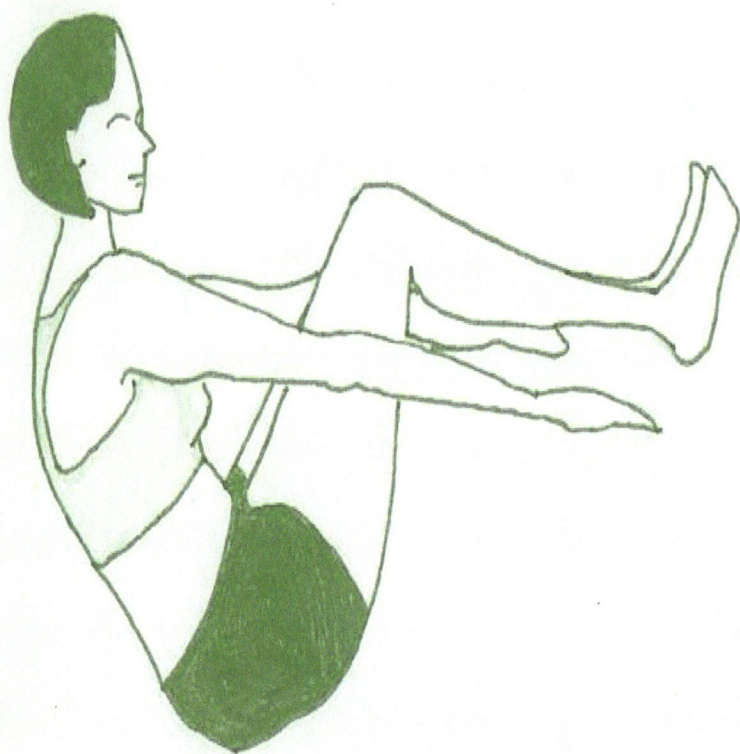

Reverse Crunches

Lie on your back, hands by your sides, feet up with and thighs perpendicular to the floor.

Place your arms by your side or rest them gently behind your head.

Roll your pelvis backward and raise your hips off the floor as you bring the knees over the chest.

Don't roll your hips backward, keep your back straight.

Hold for a two/three count as you contract your abdominals.

Return slowly to the starting position.

Perform 10-20 repetitions.

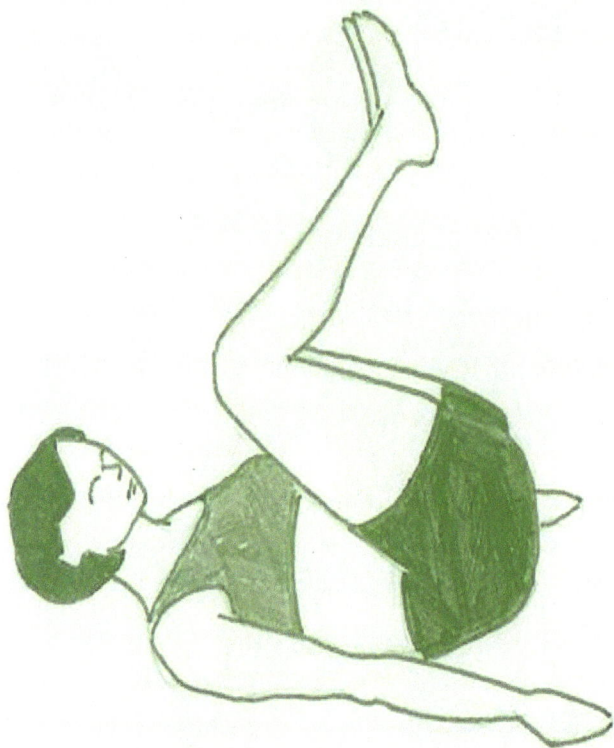

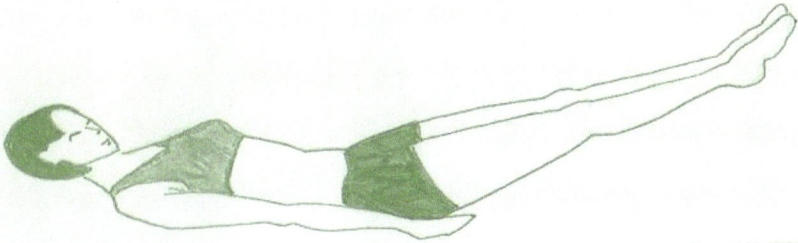

Lying Leg Lifts

Lie on the floor with arms by your sides.

Keeping the legs slightly bent and contracting the abdominals, extend the legs upward until the toes point directly overhead.

Legs should not go over the head; raise the legs until vertical.

Upper back, arms and hands are silent and remain in contact with the floor.

Slowly lower the legs until your lower back is back on the floor then lower your feet down almost to the floor to the starting position resisting on the way down.

Stay in control, don't swing the legs

As you become more comfortable with the movement, you can increase resistance by holding a dumbbell securely between your feet.

Perform 10-20 repetitions.

Jackknife Crunches

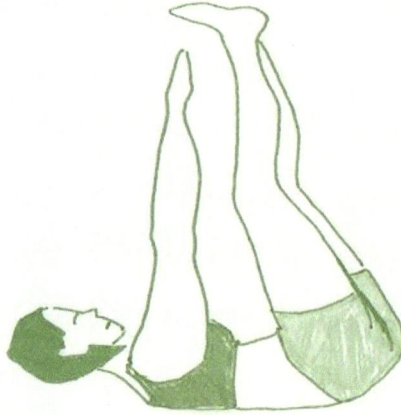

Lie on the floor with your arms extended behind your head and your legs extended upward.

First, extend your upper arms above your head.

From this position, curl your torso forward and reach your hands toward your toes.

Hold at the top of the movement, contract your abdominals for a two to three second count, then lower slowly to the starting position and repeat.

Develop a smooth rhythm without pausing between reps.

Perform 10-20 repetitions.

Hanging Leg Raises

Hang from a bar with your legs straight down.

Bend your legs and keep them bent and relaxed throughout the exercise.

Use your abdominal muscles to raise your legs toward your shoulders by flexing your waist.

DO NOT SWING.

Hold this contracted position for a slow count of one to two seconds.

Return slowly to the starting position.

You can also raise your knees to one side of the body to work your obliques.

Raise your feet higher during each repetition.

Perform 10-20 repetitions.

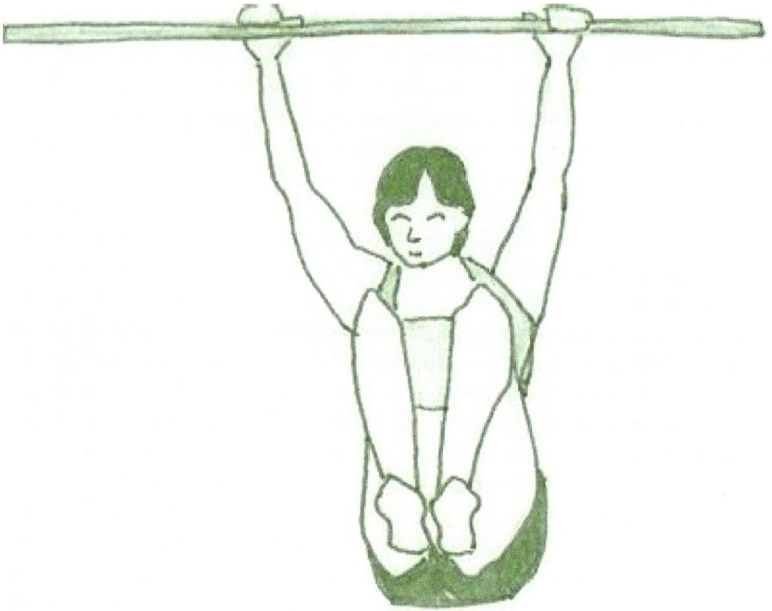

Obliques

1. Bicycle Kicks

2. Seated Trunk Twists

3. Weighted Dumbbell Side Bends

4. Alternate Heel Touchers

5. Oblique Crunches on the Floor

6. Bent-Over Twist

7. Lying Side Leg Raises

8. Russian Twist

Bicycle Kicks

Lie on your back with your hands behind your head.

Raise your legs so the lower legs are just above parallel to the floor and thighs are perpendicular to the floor.

Bring your left elbow toward your right side and draw your right knee in to meet it.

Squeeze your abs as you curl up actually rotating your shoulder as you move the elbow across your body.

Move as far as you can toward the right knee without forcing.

Switch sides and keep your movements slow and controlled as you continue the motion back and forth.

Perform 10-20 repetitions on each side.

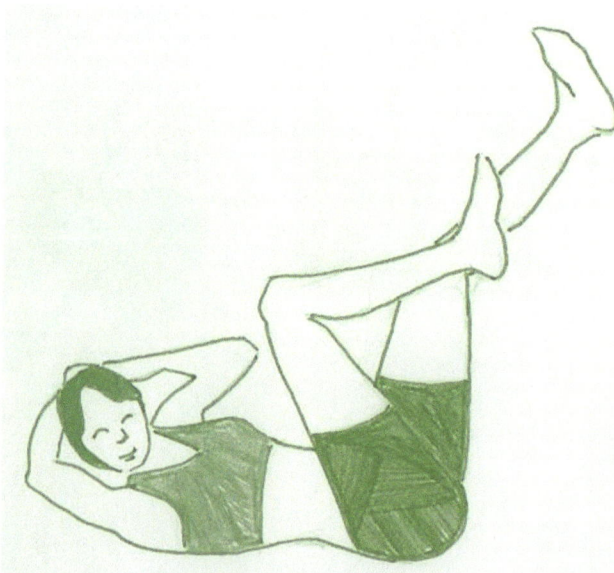

Seated Trunk Twists

Sit on the edge of the chair with the feet on the floor for support.

Hold a broomstick or bar on the shoulders using a wide grip.

Contract your abdominals and use your obliques to twist your torso to the left as far as comfortably possible.

Next, twist to the right as far as you can.

Do not jerk this movement. Keep your movements slow and controlled.

Perform 10-20 repetitions on each side.

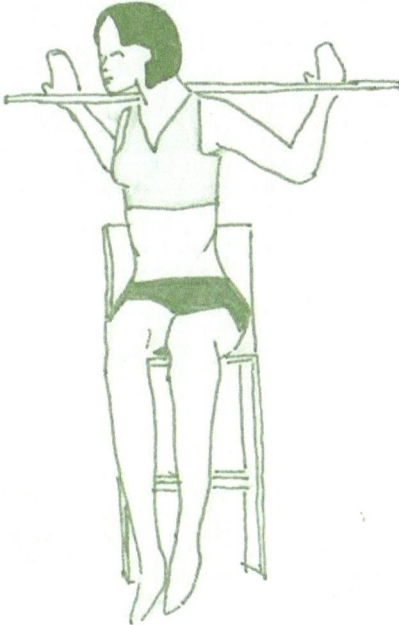

Weighted Dumbbell Side Bends

Stand tall about shoulder width apart with a dumbbell in your right hand and palms facing inwards.

Contract your abdominals and with you left hand on your waist and straight back, bend to the right as far as you can then bend to the left as far as you can.

As you bend, hips and knees remain stationary.

Don't swing. Let the waist do the work. Squeeze the obliques each time you move your torso.

Change the weight to the other hand and repeat.

Perform 25 repetitions on each side.

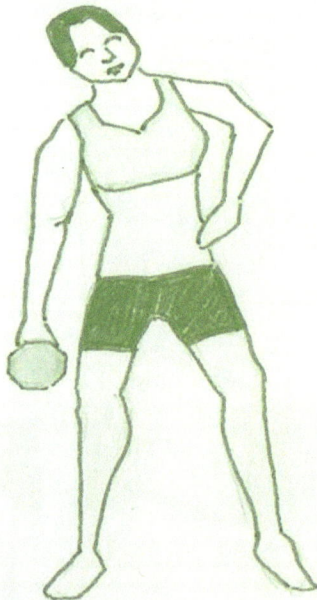

Alternate Heel Touchers

Lie on the floor and bend your knees and keep your feet about shoulder width apart.

Keep your arms at your sides, palms down.

With your lower back pressed flat against the ground, curl forward and up, extend the right arm to touch the left heel.

Head remains neutral, use the abdominals to push forward.

Hold for a second or two, and then slowly return to the starting position.

Alternate touching your right heel then left.

Perform 10-20 repetitions on both sides.

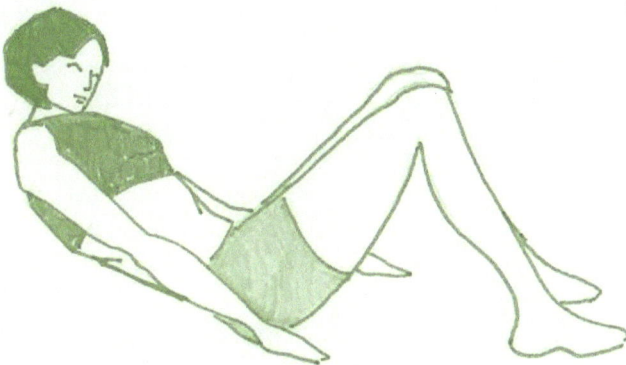

Oblique Crunches on the Floor

Lie on your right side with legs on top of each other and knees slightly bent.

Cross your right ankle over the left.

Place your left hand behind your head.

Raise your left shoulder blade without hunching the shoulders and bring the left elbow toward the right thigh as you twist your torso.

Use your obliques to crunch up.

Squeeze your abs for a two to three count then slowly lower and repeat.

Perform 10-20 repetitions on each side.

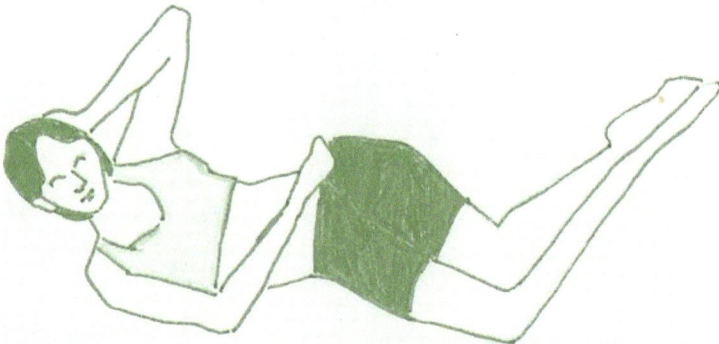

Bent-Over Twist

Stand with your feet shoulder width apart.

With a broomstick or bar at your shoulders and contracted abdominals, bend your torso at the waist so you are almost parallel to the floor. Only go as far as you can as you twist your right shoulder to the left foot.

Rotate the body through as you keep the abdominals contracted and twist your left shoulder to your right foot.

Perform 25 rotations.

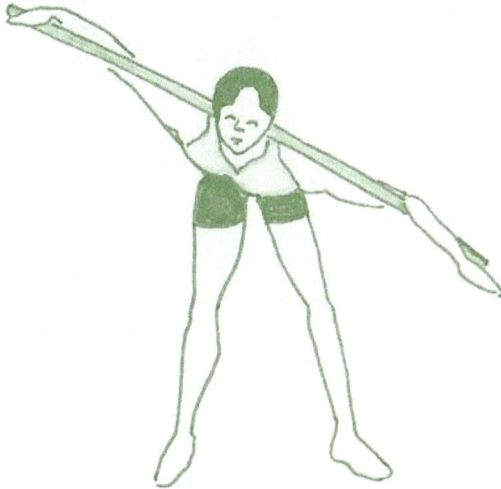

Lying Side Leg Raises

Lie on your left side with a slight bend in the knees.

Support yourself with your elbow.

Squeeze the abdominals and use your obliques to raise your right leg as high as you can.

Hold and contract.

Lower your right leg back to the starting position.

Remember to keep the legs straight as you perform this exercise.

Switch sides. Raise your left leg as high as you can.

Perform 10-20 repetitions on each side.

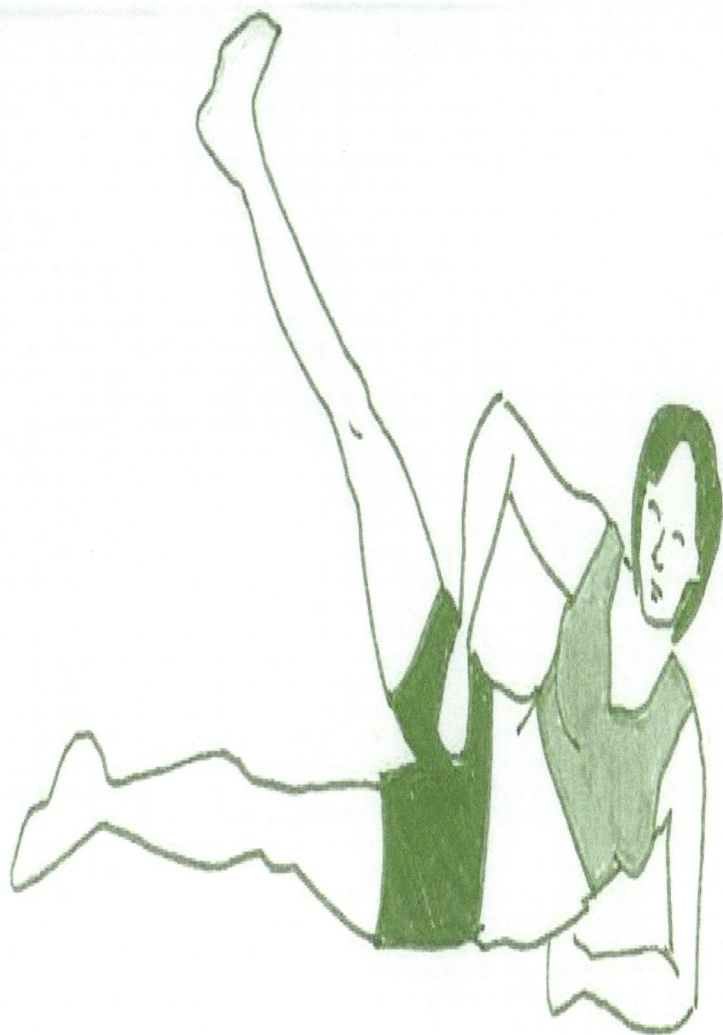

Russian Twist

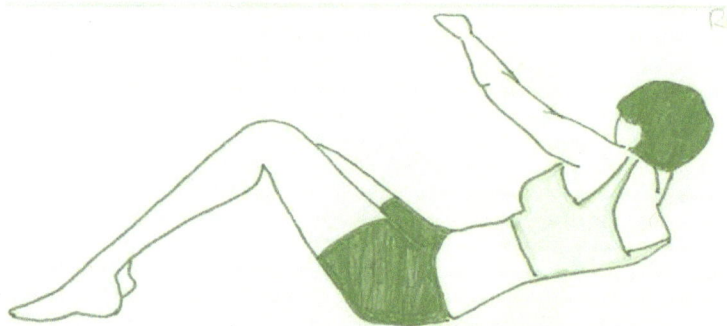

Sit on the floor with knees bent and legs extended outward.

Press your heels to the floor.

Toes are pointed upward.

Clasp your hands together and place mid-way of the body.

Lean back and contract the abs.

Contract the abdominals, pulling the navel to your spine and twist the body slowly to the right as far as possible. Knees remain bent as you focus on rotating the entire upper body. Your head should follow the arms and shoulders as you rotate the body.

Go as far as you comfortably can without compromising your back.

Pause and hold for a two to three second count.

Inhale deeply, return to center and exhale as you twist to the left side following the same guidelines.

Perform 10-20 repetitions on each side.

SIMPLE UPPER/LOWER AB EXERCISES

1. Pelvic Tilt

2. Stomach Tightener

3. Tuck Crunch

Pelvic Tilt

Lie on your back with feet shoulder-width apart.

Flatten your lower back to the floor.

Lift your lower torso upwards.

Keep the abdominals contracted.

Lower and repeat.

Perform 10-20 repetitions.

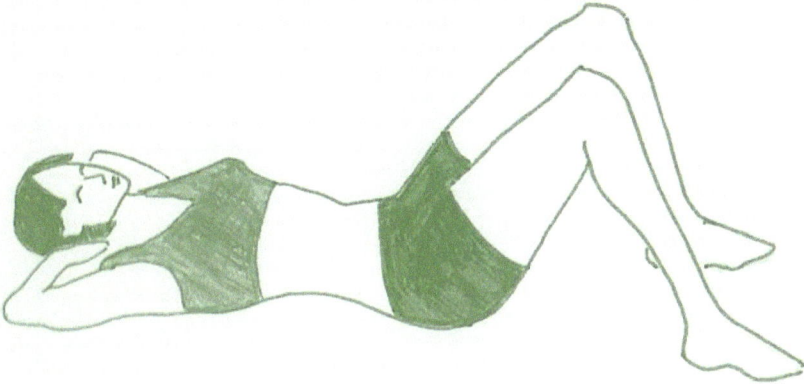

Stomach Tightener

Stand upright and place your hand on your hips.

Exhale deeply.

Inhale, expand your chest and pull the abdominals in as much as possible.

Hold the contraction for 6 counts.

Perform 10-20 repetitions.

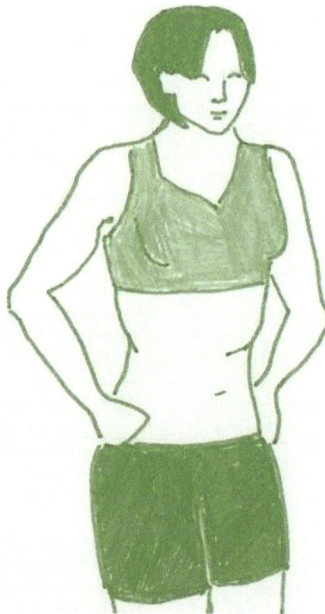

Tuck Crunch

Lie on the floor with your hands either crossed over your chest or behind your head.

Bend your knees and hips to form right angles.

Keep your lower legs parallel to the floor.

Cross your feet and lift your shoulder blades off the floor as you contract your abdominals and crunch forward.

Slowly return to the starting position.

Perform 10-20 repetitions.

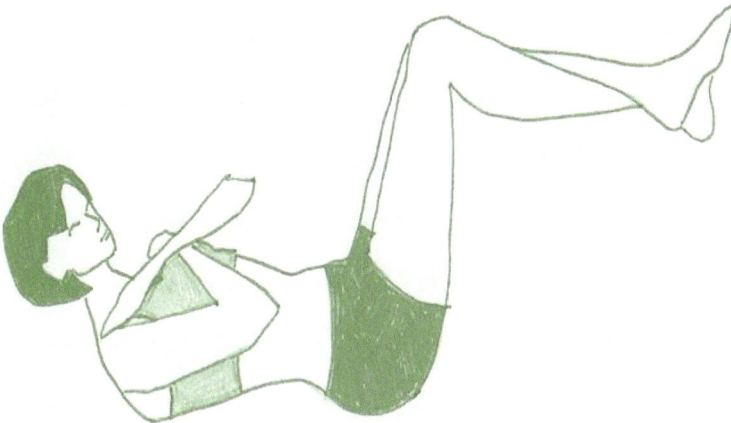

	SLOW AND STEADY – SAMPLE WORKOUT PROGRAM// WEEK OF _____			
	Upper	*Lower*	*Obliques*	✓
SUN	REST			
MON	REST			
TUES	♦ CRUNCH LEGS ON EXERCISE BALL ♦ CROSSOVER CRUNCHES ♦ FROG CRUNCHES	♦ LYING LEG LIFTS ♦ KNEE-UPS ♦ REVERSE CRUNCHES	♦ ALTERNATE HEEL TOUCHERS ♦ BICYCLE KICKS	
WED	♦ BASIC AB CRUNCH ♦ CRUNCH HANDS OVERHEAD	♦ SCISSOR KICKS ♦ HANGING LEG RAISES	♦ DUMBBELL SIDE BEND ♦ BENT-OVER TWIST ♦ OBLIQUE CRUNCHES ON THE FLOOR	
THUR	REST			
FRI	♦ WEIGHTED BALL CRUNCHES ♦ TWISTED BALL CRUNCHES ♦ CROSSOVER CRUNCHES	♦ JACKNIFE CRUNCHES ♦ LYING LEG LIFTS ♦ LEG PULL-IN	♦ SEATED TRUNK TWISTS ♦ LYING SIDE LEG RAISES	
SAT	♦ STRAIGHT LEG CRUNCHES ♦ CRUNCH LEGS ON EXERCISE BALL	♦ REVERSE CRUNCHES ♦ KNEE-UPS	♦ RUSSIAN TWIST ♦ ALTERNATE HEEL TOUCHERS ♦ DUMBBELL SIDE BEND	

Train Hard!
You will love the results in a few short weeks

www.ingramcontent.com/pod-product-compliance
Lightning Source LLC
Chambersburg PA
CBHW041221270326
41933CB00001B/4